"HELP!"

Grolier Enterprises Inc. offers a varied selection of both
adult and children's book racks. For details on ordering,
please write: Grolier Enterprises Inc., Sherman Turnpike,
Danbury, CT 06816 Attn: Premium Department

CREDITS

Producer
  Ron Berry

Editor
  Orly Kelly

What to do
when your mom or dad says ...

"HELP!"

By
JOY BERRY

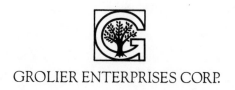

GROLIER ENTERPRISES CORP.

Has anyone ever said to you...

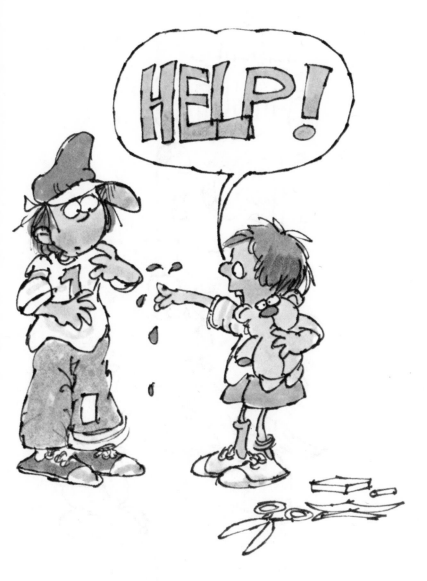

Whenever someone asks you for help, do you ever wonder...

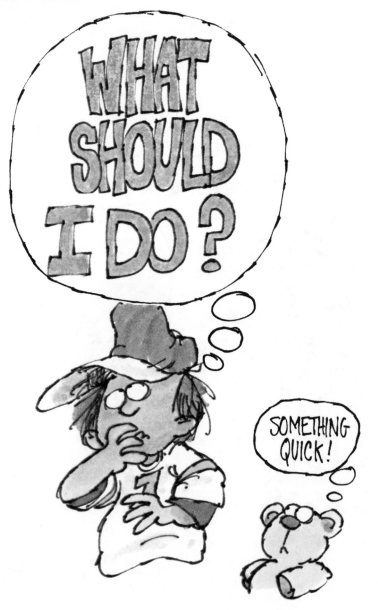

If any of this sounds familiar to you, you're going to **love** this book.

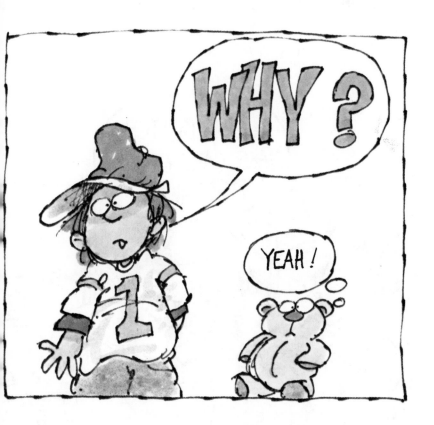

Because it will tell you exactly what to do in case of an emergency.

Sometimes during your childhood you might be involved in an emergency. An emergency is something that happens suddenly and needs attention right away.

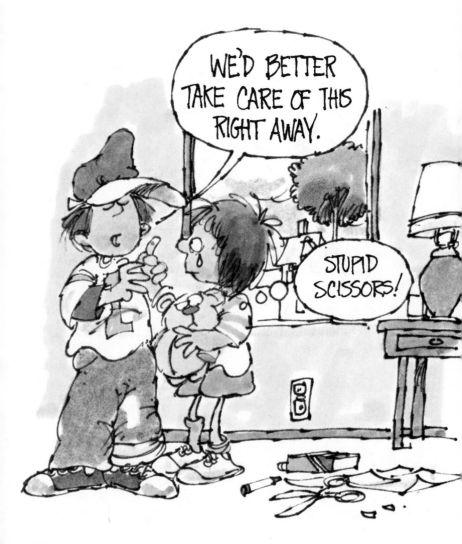

You will be able to handle some emergencies on your own, but you may need help handling others.

HANDLING MINOR EMERGENCIES

Some emergencies are minor emergencies. This means that they are not as serious as others. Usually you will be able to handle minor emergencies on your own.

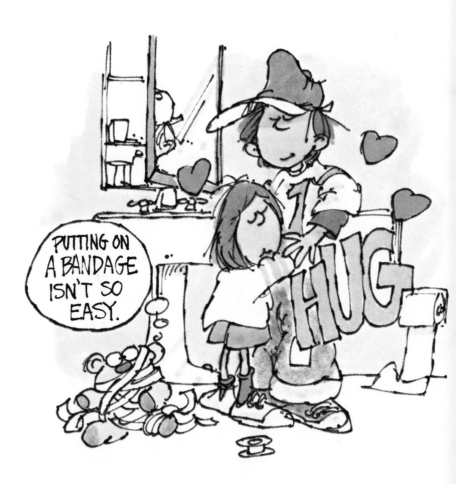

When a minor emergency happens, you should:

1. Respect it. This means you should realize that it could become a bigger problem if it is not treated properly.

2. Be conscientious. This means you should be absolutely sure that what you are doing is right, and then you should do it carefully and correctly.

3. Get help if you are frightened or if you aren't sure about what to do.

BLEEDING

To stop a wound from bleeding, put a clean gauze or cloth over the wound. (Put your clean, bare hand over the wound if you don't have any gauze or cloth.)

Then put your hand over the gauze or cloth and press firmly until you're sure the bleeding has stopped.

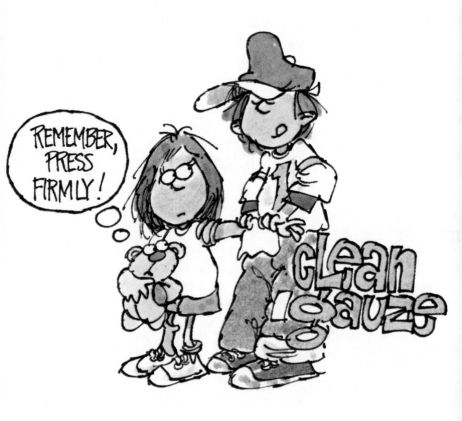

Bandage the wound firmly, but not too tightly. If you can, raise the wound above the level of the person's heart.

Any bleeding that is severe or can't be stopped needs attention right away by a person with medical training.

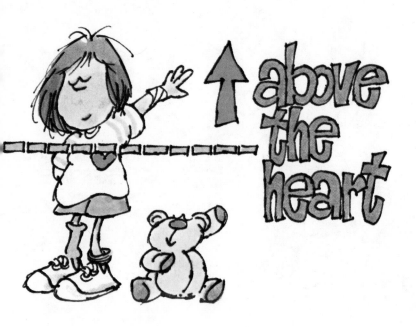

BLEEDING IN THE MOUTH

If there is bleeding in the mouth, put a small piece of clean gauze or cloth on the area that is bleeding and apply pressure until the bleeding has stopped.

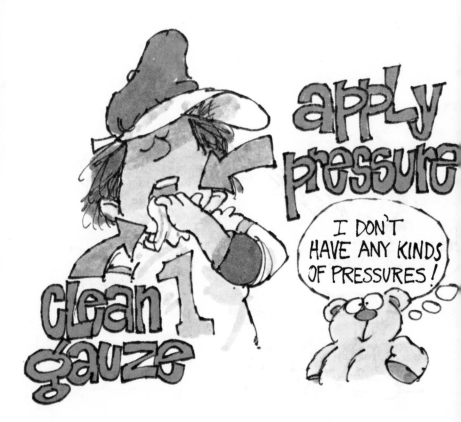

BLEEDING FROM THE NOSE

If a person has a nosebleed, he or she should breathe through the mouth while you gently pinch the nose closed for about five minutes and then apply a cold compress.

If the bleeding does not stop, pack clean gauze, cotton, or tissue in the nostril and gently pinch the nose closed for about ten minutes.

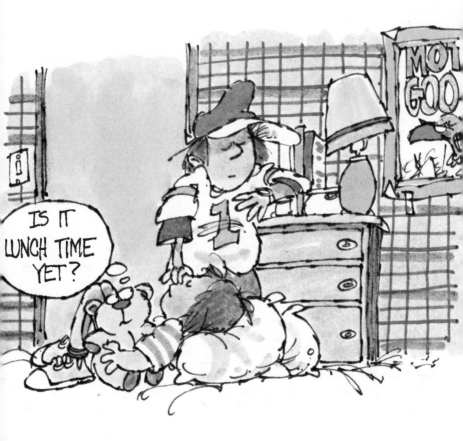

BLISTERS

If a person has a blister, do not break it open because germs can get in. The fluid inside the blister helps the skin to heal quickly. Wash the area gently with soap and water and cover it with a clean bandage.

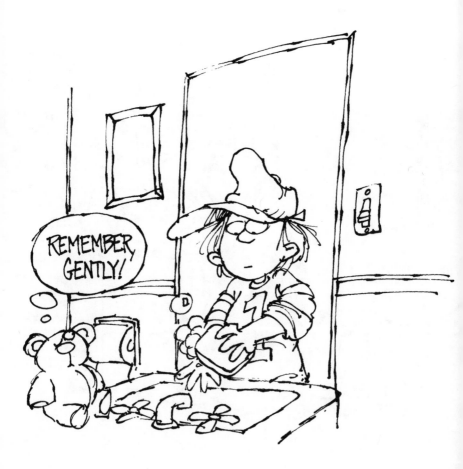

BRUISES

To care for bruises, put a cold compress on the bruised area right away.

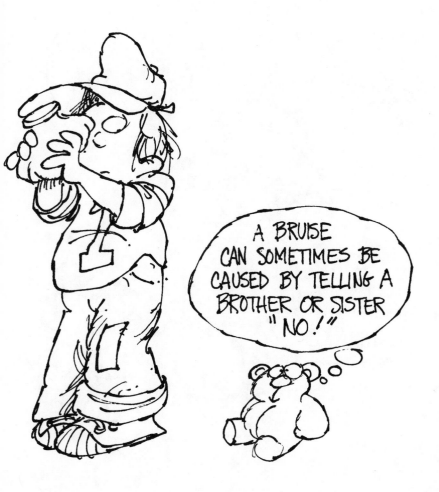

A BRUISE CAN SOMETIMES BE CAUSED BY TELLING A BROTHER OR SISTER "NO!"

BUMPS

If a person gets bumped in the head, put a cold compress on the bump. It will help the swelling go down.

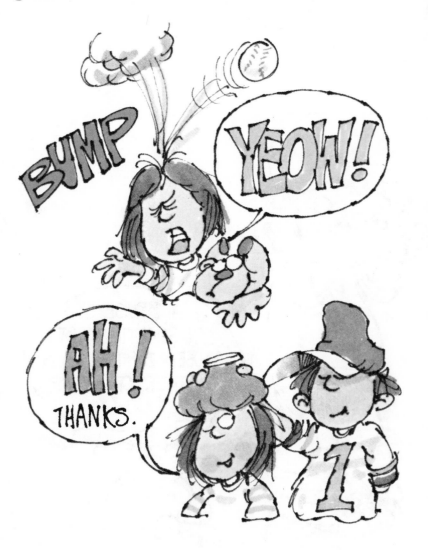

Head injuries can be very serious, even if they're small.

If the person vomits, becomes drowsy, dizzy, sweaty or pale, or if the black centers of the eyes become different sizes, he or she might have a concussion, and you need to get medical help immediately.

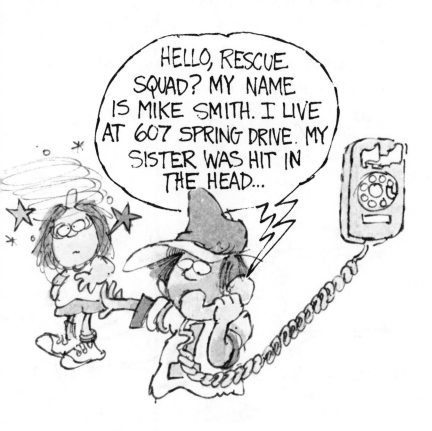

BURNS CAUSED BY CHEMICALS

If a person is burned by a chemical, immediately flush the area with plenty of cool water.

Have the person keep the burned area under cool running water for about five minutes or until it is certain that all of the chemical has been washed away. Blot the area dry with a sterile gauze or cloth and then cover it loosely with a bandage that will not stick to the burn.

If possible, raise the burned area above the level of the person's heart.

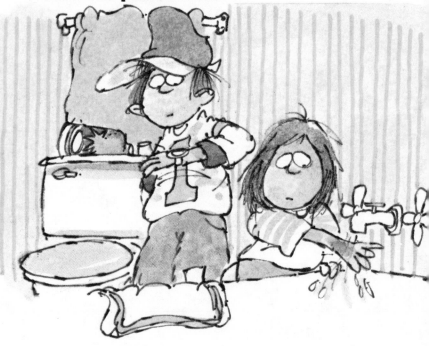

BURNS CAUSED BY HEAT

Treat the burned area with cold running water for 20 to 30 minutes until the pain goes away. (Don't use ice or ice water.)

Then gently dry and bandage the burn the same way you would a chemical burn.

Do not wash a burn, break the blisters, or use ointment or petroleum jelly on it. If a burn is serious, get medical help right away.

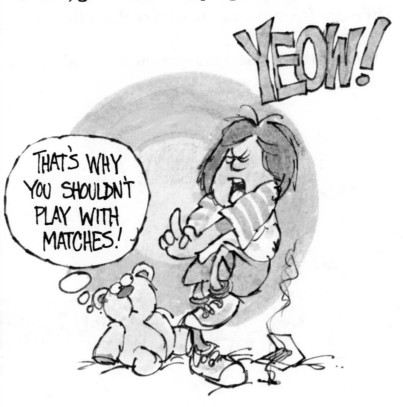

BURNS CAUSED BY THE COLD (FROSTBITE)

Frostbite occurs when part of the body starts to freeze in cold weather.

If frostbite happens, do not rub the frostbitten area. Instead, put it in lukewarm water until it is warm.

Do not use hot water.

Then dry the area gently with a clean towel.

If the frostbite is serious, get medical help right away.

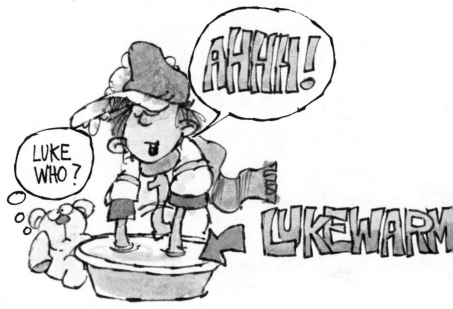

BURNS CAUSED BY THE SUN (SUNBURN)

If a person has a sunburn, bathe the sunburned area with vinegar and cover it with a clean, cold wet sheet or towel until the skin feels cool.

If you don't have any vinegar, bathe the area in cool water.

If the sunburn is serious, get medical help right away.

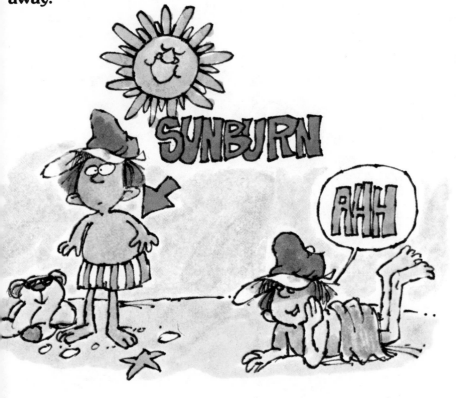

CUTS, SCRAPES, SCRATCHES AND PUNCTURES

If a person has a cut, scrape, scratch or puncture, clean the area gently but well with soap and water and apply a sterile dressing.

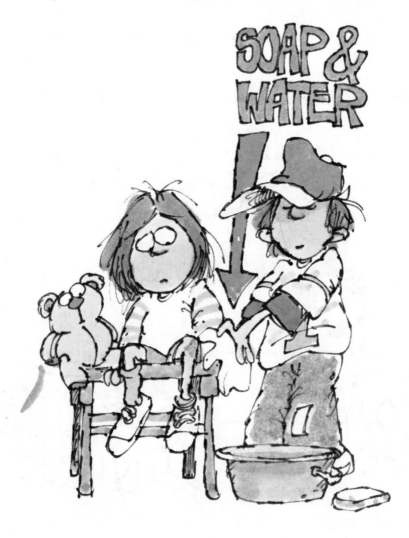

A puncture becomes infected more easily than a cut, scrape or scratch because it is hard to clean the germs out of it. This can lead to serious problems. It's a good idea to get medical help for a person who has been punctured by a dirty object, because a tetanus or booster shot may be necessary.

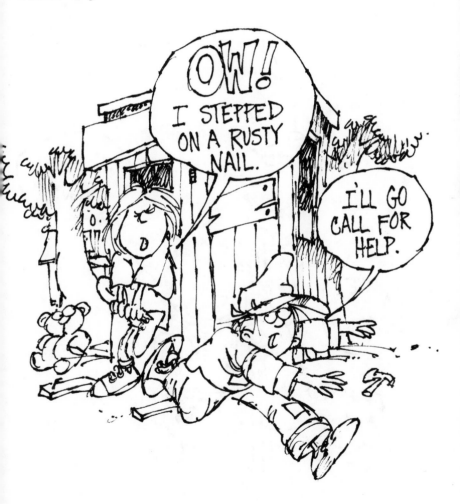

FAINTING

Persons who feel faint should lie down or sit with their heads between their legs.

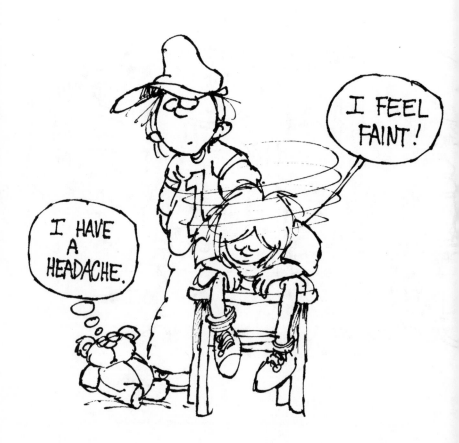

If someone faints, leave him or her lying down. Loosen any tight clothing and wipe the person's face with a cool cloth.

Do not put water on the person's face.

If the person doesn't wake up right away, get medical help immediately.

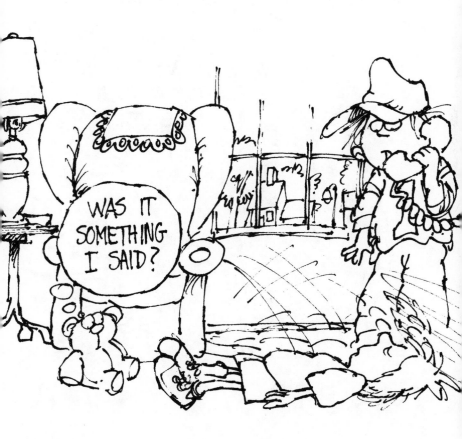

PLANT POISONING

If a person has come in contact with a poisonous plant, have the person take off any clothing that might have been touched by the plant. Then wash the person's skin with soap and water and apply rubbing alcohol. If a rash appears, put calamine lotion on it.

If the reaction to the plant poisoning becomes serious, get medical help right away.

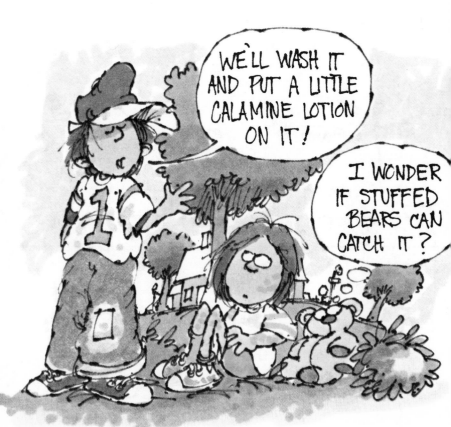

STINGS

If a person is stung by an insect, wash the sting with soap and water, soothe the area with a clean cold compress, and put calamine lotion on it.

If the person is allergic to the insect that has bitten him or her, get medical help right away. Stings can be deadly for persons who have severe allergic reactions.

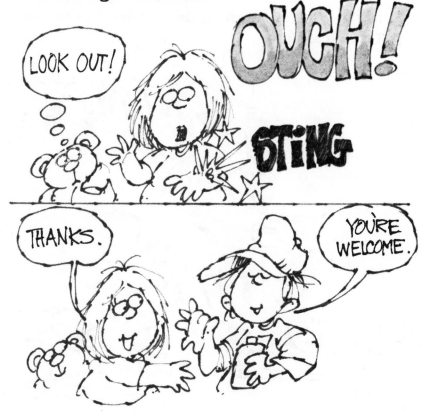

SPLINTERS

If a person gets a splinter stuck under the skin, sterilize a needle by putting it in a flame or by cleaning it off with alcohol, and use the needle to lift the skin that is over the splinter. Then slide the splinter out with the needle or pull it out with tweezers.

Clean the area gently with soap and water.

If the splinter is embedded deeply in the skin, get medical help.

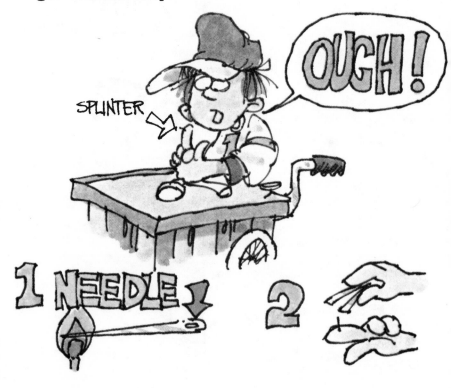

STRAINS

If a person strains a muscle by stretching or pulling it too much, apply a warm wet compress to the strained area and encourage the person to rest it.

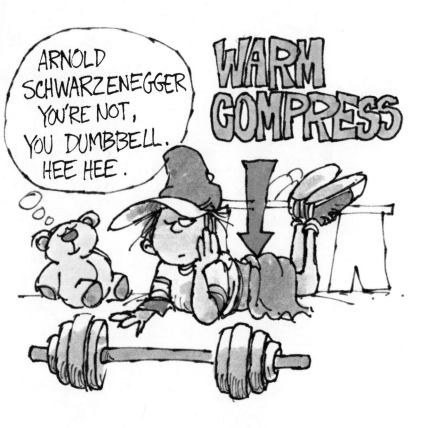

Handle minor emergencies by—

- respecting them,
- being conscientious, and
- getting help whenever necessary

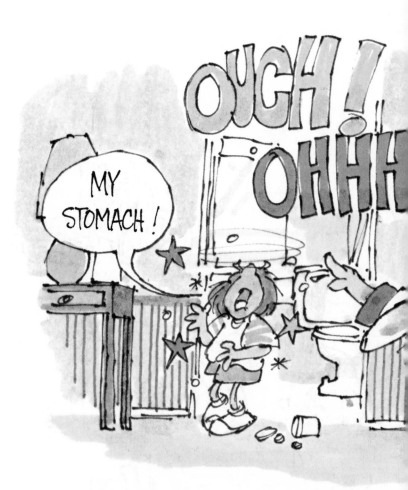

Get medical help immediately for serious injuries and illnesses, and never give or take any medication unless you are told to do so by a responsible adult.

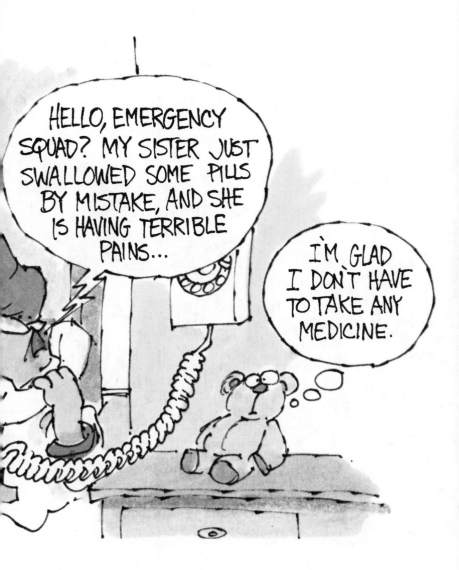

33

HANDLING MAJOR EMERGENCIES

Some emergencies are major emergencies. This means they are very serious because a person's life is in danger.

Usually you will not be able to handle major emergencies by yourself, because you won't have enough—

- strength,
- skill, or
- training.

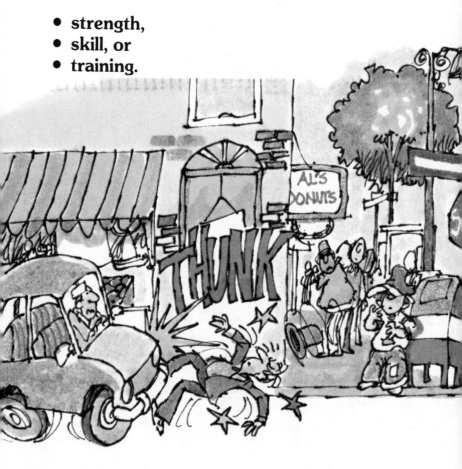

When a major emergency occurs, do not try to take care of it yourself. Get help right away!

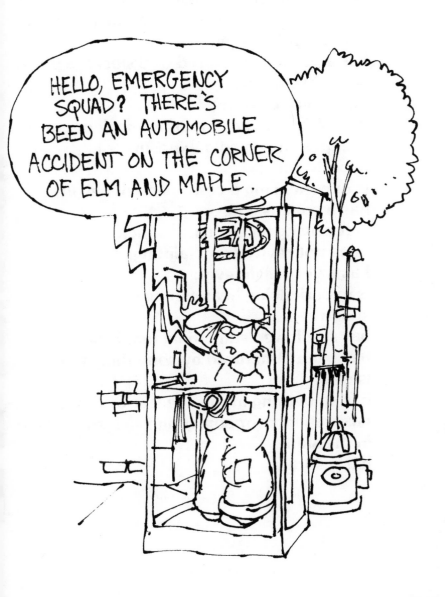

An emergency is **major** when a person:

- is having a severe allergic reaction;
- is bleeding uncontrollably;
- is bitten by a person or an animal, and the skin is broken open;
- has a broken, fractured or dislocated bone;
- is not breathing;
- has a serious burn;
- is choking or can't breathe, speak or cough;
- is experiencing cold exposure, or hypothermia;
- is experiencing a convulsion or seizure;
- has a concussion;
- is receiving an electrical shock;
- does not revive from fainting;
- has a very high fever;
- is experiencing heat exhaustion or sunstroke;
- has swallowed something that is poisonous;
- has been punctured by something that is dirty;
- has something in the eye, ear or nose;
- has a splinter or something else stuck deep in the skin;
- has a sprain.

You can never know when a major emergency is going to occur, so you need to be sure that you are in contact with an adult who can help you at all times.

This means:

1. Wherever you go, make sure there is an adult close by who can get to you immediately.
2. If you are ever left at home alone, make sure you know what adult you are to contact in case of an emergency.
3. Try always to have someone else with you when you are away from home so that if one of you needs help, the other one can get it.

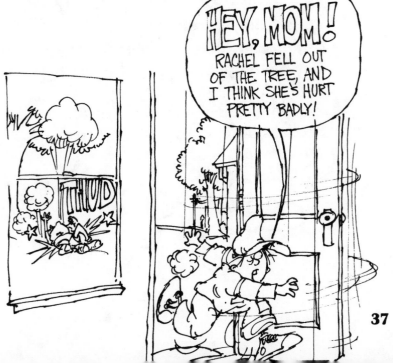

BROKEN BONES

1. Broken bones usually do not kill. Do not move the victim unless there is **immediate danger** of further injury.
2. Call for emergency help.
3. Do not try to push the broken bone back into place if it is sticking out of the skin. Do apply a moist dressing on the injury to prevent its drying out.

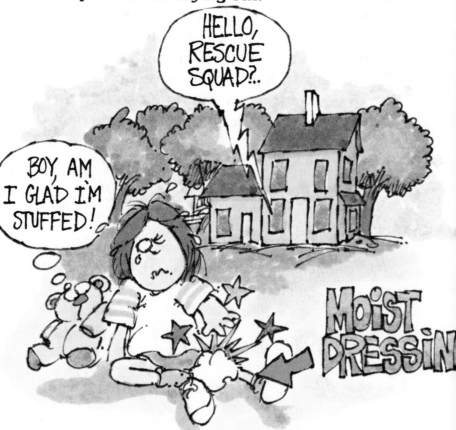

4. Do not try to straighten out a fracture. Let a doctor or a trained person do that.
5. Do not permit the victim to walk about.
6. Keep the victim calm and warm while waiting for help to arrive.

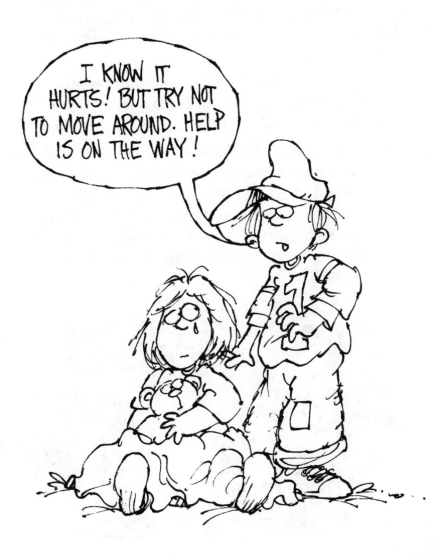

CHOKING

Anything stuck in the throat blocking the air passage can stop a person's breathing.

Do not interfere with a choking victim who can speak, cough or breathe. However, if the choking continues without lessening, call for emergency medical help.

If the victim cannot speak, cough or breath, immediately have someone call for emergency medical help while you take the following action:

1. Stand just behind and to the side of the victim, who can be standing or sitting. Support the victim with one hand on the chest. The victim's head should be lowered. Give four sharp blows between the shoulder blades. If unsuccessful, try the method described on page 43.

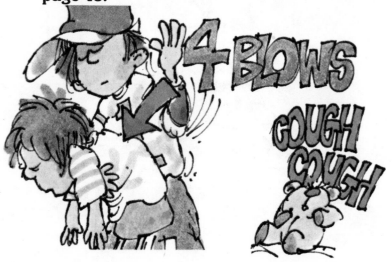

2. Stand behind the victim, who can be standing or sitting, and wrap your arms around his or her middle just above the navel. Clasp your hands together in a doubled fist and press in and up sharply in quick thrusts. Repeat several times.

If still unsuccessful, repeat four back blows and four quick thrusts until the victim is no longer choking.

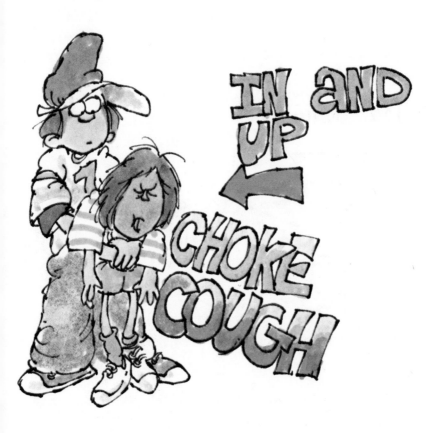

POISONING

Small children are most often the victims of accidental poisoning. If a child has swallowed or is suspected to have swallowed any substance that might be poisonous, assume the worst—take action.

Call your Poison Control Center. If none is in your area, call your Fire Department Rescue Squad. Keep suspect item and container with you to show to rescue squad when it arrives.

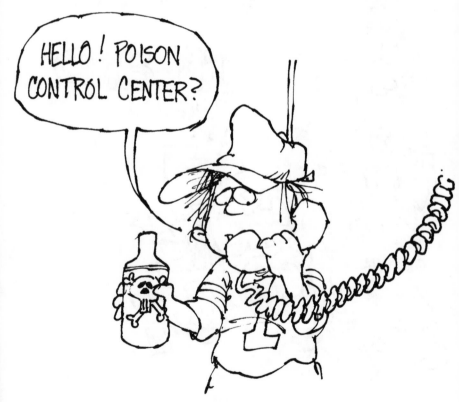

If the victim is vomiting, roll him or her over onto the left side so that the person will not choke on what is brought up.

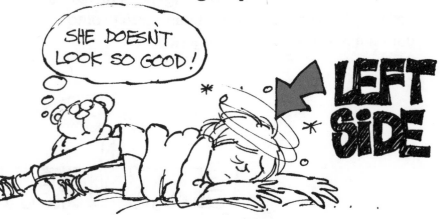

Be prepared. Keep the Poison Control Center and Fire Department Rescue Squad numbers near your telephone.

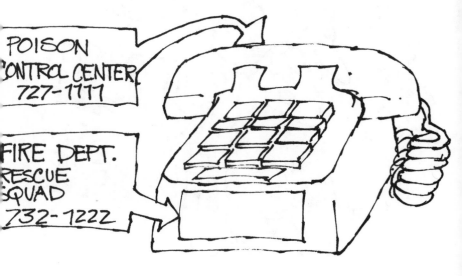

43

HANDLING NATURAL DISASTERS

You may experience an emergency caused by nature. There are things you can do to protect yourself in this kind of emergency.

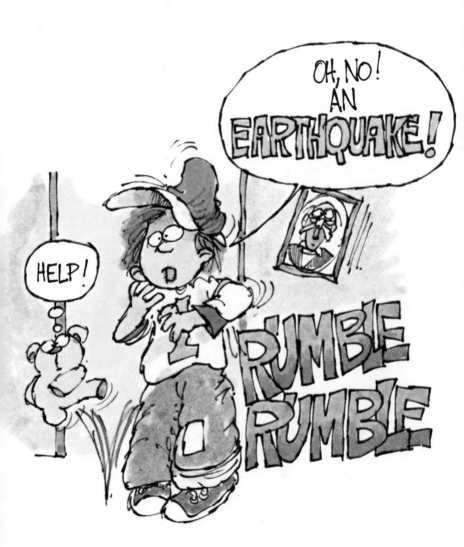

EMERGENCY PROCEDURES FOR EARTHQUAKES

If you are indoors, stay there. Cover your face and head while standing in a doorway, or curl up under a table or desk, making sure your head and face are covered. Stay in this position until the earthquake is over. Stay clear of windows.

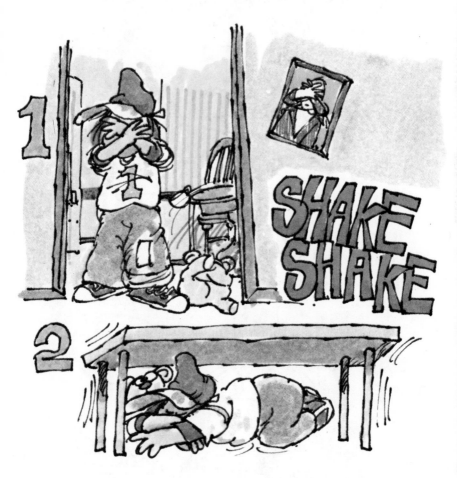

EMERGENCY PROCEDURE FOR LIGHTNING, RAIN AND WINDSTORMS

Find shelter immediately, and stay inside until the storm is over. Note: never stand under a tree in an electrical storm.

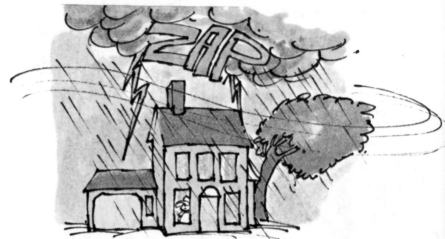

EMERGENCY PROCEDURE FOR FLOODS

If you can, leave the flooded area immediately. If you are not able to get out, go to the highest point you can find and stay there until you are rescued.

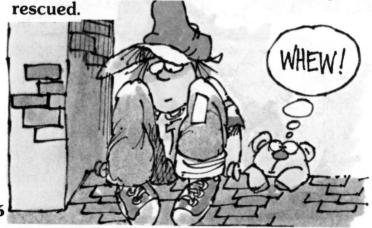

EMERGENCY PROCEDURE FOR
HURRICANES AND TORNADOES

Find shelter in a cellar or basement, and stay there until the hurricane or tornado is over.

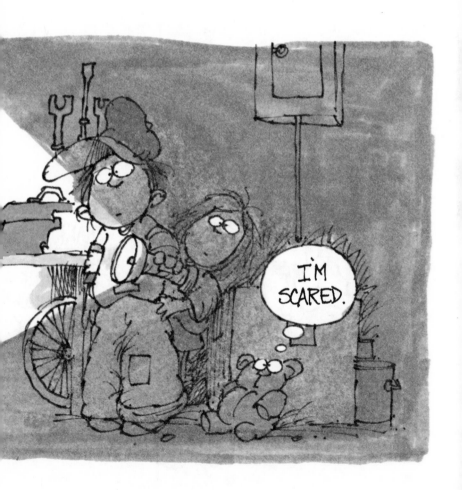

THE END of not knowing what to do when someone needs help!

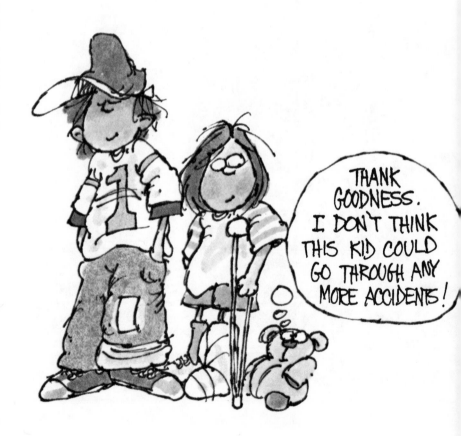